WALL PILATES WORKOUT GUIDE FOR WEIGHT LOSS

A step by step low impact resistance guide to tone glutes, shape

Abs improve muscle strength, reduce weight strengthen core

Achieve flexibility and balance, suitable for beginners

Intermediate and seniors

BONUS

Sample Meal Plans

Doris A. Freema

Copyright

Disclaimer

It is important to note that the information provided in this publication is for General informational purposes only. We have made every effort to ensure that the Information is accurate and up-to-date, however, we cannot guarantee its Completeness, accuracy, reliability, suitability, or availability. Any reliance you Place on such information is at your own risk. The exercises, practices, and Recommendations provided are not a substitute for professional advice, diagnosis, Or treatment.

Always consult with a qualified health Provider with any questions you may have

Regarding a medical condition. We cannot be held liable for any injury, damage, or

Loss incurred as a direct or indirect consequence of the use or application of any

Content presented in this publication. It is recommended to consult with a qualified

Loss incurred as a direct or indirect consequence of the use or application of any

Content presented in this publication. It is recommended to consult with a qualified

Professional before making any changes to your fitness, health, or lifestyle.

By using this publication, you acknowledge and agree to these terms and conditions

About the author

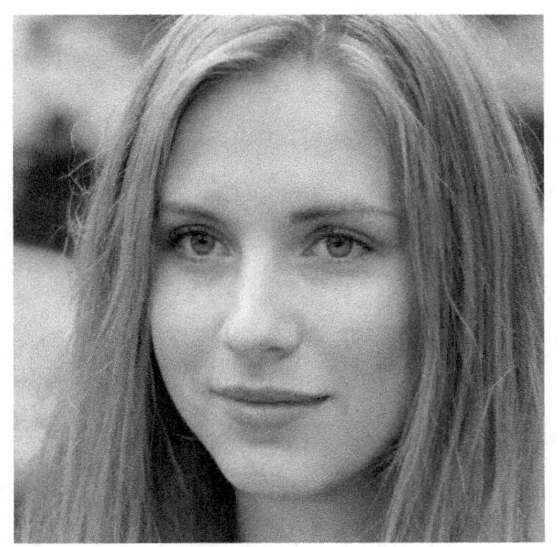

Meet the insightful mind behind the transformative guide, "Wall Pilates guide for Weight loss," the esteemed Doris A. Freema. As a dedicated advocate for women's health and fitness, Doris brings a wealth of expertise to her work, blending her passion for movement with a commitment to holistic well-being. Doris A. Freema, a certified Pilate's instructor and wellness enthusiast, embarked on her journey in the world of fitness with an ardent desire to empower women in their pursuit of a healthier and more balanced life. Married and rooted in a supportive family environment, Doris draws inspiration from her personal experiences in navigating the challenges and triumphs of maintaining well-being within the dynamic context of modern life. Doris's professional journey is marked by a deep dedication to the Pilates discipline. Trained under renowned Pilate's practitioners and having accumulated years of hands-on experience, she has honed her expertise in tailoring Pilate's routines to the specific needs and goals of women. Doris is recognized for her ability to seamlessly integrate Pilates into various lifestyles, making it accessible and beneficial for women at all fitness levels. What sets Doris apart is not just her technical proficiency but her holistic approach to

Health. Her philosophy revolves around the idea that true wellness extends beyond the physical aspects of exercise. In "Wall Pilates for weight loss," she delves into the mental, emotional, and spiritual dimensions of well-being, offering a comprehensive guide that resonates with the multifaceted nature of women's lives. As a woman dedicated to empowering women, Doris is not only an instructor but an advocate for the transformative power of fitness

In women's lives. Her approach recognizes and celebrates the unique strengths and challenges that women face, providing not just a fitness guide but a roadmap for embracing one's Feminine strength and resilience. Married to a supportive partner, Doris understands the delicate dance of maintaining a harmonious work-life balance. In her book, she shares personal anecdotes and strategies for women to integrate Pilates seamlessly into their daily routines, demonstrating that prioritizing health does not mean compromising on personal relationships or other life commitments. Doris's venture into writing is an extension of her commitment to reaching a wider audience. "Wall Pilates for Women" is a labor of love, a culmination of her experiences, insights, and a desire to make a lasting impact on the lives of women seeking a holistic approach to wellness. Outside the realm of Pilates, Doris is an advocate for community engagement and regularly conducts workshops, webinars, and community events to spread awareness about the benefits of mindful movement. Her warm and engaging personality has garnered her a community of followers who appreciate not just her expertise but her genuine passion for helping women thrive. Doris A. Freema is not just an author; she is a beacon of inspiration for women on their journey to wellness. Through her book, she invites readers into a transformative space where the union of physical, mental, and emotional well-being takes center stage. Doris, with her rich background, brings a unique blend of professionalism and relatability, creating a lasting impact on the landscape of women's fitness literature. As readers delve into "Wall Pilates for Weight loss," they are guided by the experienced hand and compassionate heart of an author who is not just a master of her craft but a true advocate for the flourishing health and vitality of women.

Table of content

Introduction 11

Getting started with wall Pilates..13

The Basics of Pilates 17

Wall Pilates Exercises 21

Structured Wall Pilates Workouts 25

Nutrition and Weight Loss 29

Sample Meal Plans Bonus 31

Staying motivated...35

Tips for Safe and Effective Wall Pilates 39

Conclusion..43

Your opinion matters..45

Introduction

In the peaceful town of Tranquil Ville, surrounded by calm hills and soft water sounds, Emma lived. She was a strong-hearted woman who wanted to change herself for the better. Emma, just like many others, tried a lot of ways to lose weight. She used different methods that didn't make her happy or energized. One day, a chance encounter at her local fitness studio introduced her to a secret world of fitness that would redefine her journey: wall Pilates. This guide tells the story of Emma finding out things and what she learned during that time. It's like a guide for people who want to lose weight, but also find balance between being strong and flexible while thinking carefully about their lives. Join us in Emma's place as we show the secret goodies of Wall Pilates. This guide shows how practicing the wall and each move can help you grow better. It explains special ways of thinking that go beyond normal activities. Join Emma while she explores the heart of Pilates - a set of thought-out movements, the beat of air, and deep links between body and brain. She found out that these ideas aren't just games; they are the tools to open a healthier and more full-of-life version of oneself. This book is not just a how-to guide; it's Emma's experience which she now shares with you. Let's start together a journey driven by meaning, accuracy, and the good feeling that Wall Pilates gives.

Are you prepared to change your story?

Getting started with wall Pilates

Introduction to Wall Pilates

Welcome to the starting point of your amazing fitness trip-Wall Pilates. In this Chapter, we will go on a journey to learn about Wall Pilates. We'll discover what makes it special and how it can help you lose weight better. Using the Power of Wall to Unlock Benefits Find out how the wall can be used as a helpful and changing tool in Pilates. Find out how this help system makes your balance better, lets you line up more easily and adds a new level to your exercise routine.

Mixing Old Ways with New Ideas

Look at how classical Pilate's ideas can smoothly connect with new wall-based workouts. Get how this mix makes a whole way of exercise, going after not only your center but also the rest of your body.

Create Your Wall Pilates Area.

Making the right space is important for good Wall Pilates. Here, we'll show you how

To organize your workout area so it feels great and works well.

Choosing the Right Wall

Know what makes a good wall for your practice. If you're at home or in a gym, learn

How to use what's around for safe and fun Pilates.

Essential Equipment

Look into what basic tools are needed for Wall Pilates. We will list things like mats

And bands that can make your exercises better. These items help improve workouts

For your practice too.

Proper Body Alignment

Getting your body in the right position is very important for doing good Wall Pilates.

In this part, we'll look at why being in the right position is important and how it

Makes each exercise work better.

Finding Your Neutral Spine

Learn about a straight back and know how it works as the base for many Wall Pilates

Moves. Learn ways to spot and keep this best place during your exercise sessions.

Mindful Position and Breathing Control

Find the connection between how you sit and control your breathing. Find out how

Mindfulness is very important for getting the most from wall Pilates. It helps to make

Your   body   and   mind   connect   better.

16

The Basics of Pilates

Core Principles of Pilates

When you start doing Wall Pilates, it's very important to know the main rules. In this

Part, we'll look at the important basics that make up Pilates and help us start a healthy

Way of doing exercise.

Control and Precision

Start learning how to use your body in purposeful ways. Find out how doing each

Exercise carefully doesn't just make it better but also keeps you safe from getting

Hurt. Find out the strength of intentional, planned actions.

Centering and Core Engagement

Find out what it means to focus, which is where the main part of Pilates comes from.

Try out workouts that help your core muscles get stronger and more active. This will

Make it easier for you to stay steady on your feet.

Flow and Fluidity

Enjoy the flowing motions in Pilate's exercises. Learn how moving smoothly from

One exercise to another makes your workouts feel like a dance. This helps you

Become more graceful and quick on your feet.

Importance of Breath Control

Breath is what drives Pilates. It gives us life. In this part, we'll look at why mindful

Breathing is important and how it helps to improve your body-mind connection while doing Wall Pilates.

Diaphragmatic Breathing

Learn how to breathe properly using your diaphragm. See how matching your breath

With actions not only gives oxygen to your body, but also helps you relax and

Concentrate.

Breathe a Tool for Balance

Learn how your breath helps keep you steady. Learn ways to use your breath smartly,

Making a good balance between breathing and muscle activity.

Connecting Mind and Body in Pilates

Pilates is more than just physical exercise; it's a mindful activity. This part looks at

How your mind and body are deeply connected, making your Wall Pilates more like

A whole journey of understanding yourself.

Mindful Awareness

Develop awareness as you do each exercise. Learn ways to focus all your attention

On the now, creating a stronger link with your body.

Visualization and Positive Affirmations

Use power of thinking in pictures and saying positive things to help yourself. Learn

How these mind skills can make you better, increase excitement and help towards a

Happy attitude during your Wall Pilates exercise.

Wall Pilates Exercises

Welcome to the center of your Wall Pilates exercises. In this part, we will try Different activities to use the wall's help. These make your muscles and body Healthier. Every exercise is made to connect your center, start muscle parts, and add a new part to your workout plan.

Warm-up Exercises

Neck and Shoulder Rolls

Start your Wall Pilates workout with easy neck and shoulder rolls. These actions Take away stress, make blood flow better and get your top half ready for the next. Activities

Ankle Rolls

Start moving your lower body by rolling your ankles. Get better at stretching and Loosen up your joints, this will help you do the coming activities easier.

Spinal Flexion and Extension

Use your back muscles with slow bends and stretches. This easy exercise helps you

Move better, boosts blood flow and prepares your middle for the tougher Pilates

Moves.

Core Strengthening Exercises

Sit against a wall and rock your hips forwards and back. This can help correct

Misaligned bones in the pelvis that may be causing pain or stiffness.

Use the power of the wall to make your core stronger. The wall sit with pelvic tilts

Makes your lower tummy and leg muscles stronger. It helps make you steady too!

Leg Lifts

Make your stomach muscles stronger with leg lifts. Using the wall for help, this

Exercise tests your lower tummy muscles. It also helps with balance and control of

Movement.

Plank Variations

Try different types of planks against the wall. These workouts help make your

belly

Strong but also workout your arms, shoulders and back muscles. They give a

Complete body exercise.

Lower Body Focus

Wall Squats

Look at how your legs work with the wall when you do a squat against it. Use only

These 200 words or more in English: Explore and investigate the relationship

Between your leg muscles, bones, and tendons as they connect to other parts of your

Body during wall squats. This exercise helps don't just make them stronger but also

Improves balance for overall daily living this exercise for the lower body makes your

Thighs and butt stronger. It also helps you to keep good posture when doing it.

Hamstring Curls

Do wall hamstring curls to make your leg muscles strong and keep knees stable. This

Activity mixes strength and flexibility for a good lower body training.

Upper Body Engagement

Arm Circles

Improve your arm strength and shoulder flexibility by doing wall-assisted circles

With arms. This workout uses your upper body while adding the balancing help of a wall.

Wall Push-Ups

Learn how to do wall push-ups for strength in your upper body. This activity works

On your chest, shoulders and arms while making sure the movements are steady and

Easy.

Structured Wall Pilates Workouts

In this part, we'll show you how to do Wall Pilates workouts in a set way that are Made for different fitness levels. These activities are made to slowly test your body, keeping the rules of control, accuracy and careful focus. If you're new, still learning or a strong fan of exercise - these workouts will help make your muscles stronger, improve being bendy and support when losing weight.

Beginner's Wall Pilates Workout

Week 1

Warm-up (5 minutes):

Neck and shoulder rolls

Ankle rolls

Spinal flexion and extension

Core Strengthening (10 minutes):

Sit on the wall and do pelvic tilts (do it 2 times, each time for ten repetitions).

Raise leg (do twice, 10 times each leg)

Plank next to the wall (2 sets of 15 seconds)

Lower Body Focus (8 minutes):

Wall sit (2 sets of 12 repetitions)

Leg curls (2 sets of 10 times each leg)

Cool Down (5 minutes):

Easy stretching focusing on big muscle groups.

Week 2

Grow by increasing one group for each exercise.

Week 3

Add changes and make each exercise last longer.

Intermediate Wall Pilates Workout

Week 1

Warm-up (5 minutes):

Neck and shoulder rolls

Ankle rolls

Spinal flexion and extension

Core Strengthening (15 minutes):

Sit on a wall with movements in your hips (do this three times for 12 seconds each).

Move your legs up and down 3 times, doing it for each leg twelve ways.

Plank changes (3 sets of 20 seconds each)

Lower Body Focus (10 minutes):

Wall squats (3 sets of 15 repetitions)

Leg curls (3 sets of 12 times each leg Upper Body Engagement (8 minutes):

Do arm circles (2 sets of 15 times each way) to stretch out your arms.

Do 3 sets of 12 wall push-ups.

Cool Down (5 minutes):

Comprehensive stretching routine

Week 2

Make it harder by adding little weight or moving to tougher versions.

Week 3

Push yourself to go for longer times and add more repetitions.

Advanced Wall Pilates Workout

Week 1

Warm-up (5 minutes):

Neck and shoulder rolls

Ankle rolls

Spinal flexion and extension

Core Strengthening (20 minutes):

Do pelvic tilts while sitting against a wall (4 sets of 15 times) with rests in between.

Lift your leg (do 4 groups of 15 times for each leg).

Planks with different changes (do 4 sets of 30 seconds each time)

Lower Body Focus (15 minutes):

Do wall squats (4 times with 20 steps each)

15 times for each leg on 4 sets of hamstring curls.

Upper Body Engagement (12 minutes)

Do 3 sets of arm circles, moving in both directions. Do each direction for a total of 20 times.

Push-ups against a wall (4 sets of 15 reps)

Cool Down (5 minutes):

Advanced stretching routine

Week 2

Add fancy changes, like single-sided exercises and extra strength work.

Week 3

Keep pushing yourself to do it for longer times, work harder and figure out more

Difficult patterns.

29

Nutrition and Weight Loss

On your journey with Wall Pilates, it's very important to eat well along with doing the exercises. Stick to foods that will give you good health. This part looks at how good food and losing weight go together. It gives information about careful eating, planning your meals, and choosing what you eat that fits with getting fitter.

Why Nutrition is Key for Weight Loss

Understanding Caloric Balance

Understand the idea of caloric balance and how it affects weight loss. Find out how

To eat the right amount of food and burn it off using Wall Pilates or other exercises.

Nutrient-Rich Foods

Look at why nutrient-filled foods matter. Find out how adding different types of Vitamins, minerals and big food groups helps not just in losing weight but also being healthy overall.

Pilates and Dietary Synergy

Fueling Your Workouts

Find the best food eating plans before and after your workout. Learn what food you Eat to get the most energy, make Wall Pilates better and help fast recovery.

Hydration

Learn how important it is to drink water when doing Pilates and losing weight. Learn how drinking enough water helps your digestion, speeds up metabolism and Keeps you healthy in general.

Sample Meal Plans Bonus

Breakfast

Eggs with spinach and tomatoes

Whole-grain toast

Kids love fresh fruit like berries or an apple.

Mid-Morning Snack:

Greek yogurt with a few almonds added in.

Lunch

Lightly cooked chicken or tofu salad with different types of leaves, tasty red

Tomatoes, cucumber and simple vinegar sauce for dressing.

Cook quinoa or brown rice as a side dish.

Afternoon Snack

Sliced bell peppers with hummus

Dinner

Bake salmon or a protein food from plants. If you prefer, choose plant based proteins

Instead of the baked fish.

Steamed broccoli and quinoa

Olive oil dressing on a salad with green vegetables.

Evening Snack (if needed)

Cottage cheese with some nuts added on top.

Vegetarian Delight

Breakfast

Banana and spinach smoothie made with almond milk, plus a scoop of protein

Powder added in.

Whole-grain toast with avocado

Mid-Morning Snack

Handful of mixed berries

Lunch

Lentil and vegetable soup

Quinoa or whole-grain pita alongside the main dish

Afternoon Snack:

Yogurt with honey and walnuts from Greece.

Dinner

Cooked veggie sticks (bell peppers, zucchini and cherry tomatoes)

Lemon-tahini dressing with chickpea salad.

Evening Snack (if needed):

Sliced apple with nut butter

High-Protein Day

Breakfast

Breakfast made with eggs, cooked mushrooms, onions and feta cheese.

Whole-grain English muffin

Mid-Morning Snack:

Protein shake with almond milk

Staying motivated

Starting a health journey with Wall Pilates to lose weight needs commitment and

Patience. This part is about tips and ideas that will help you stay excited throughout

Your Pilates exercises, making sure you keep going strong always.

Setting Realistic Goals

Understanding SMART Goals

Learn why it is important to make clear, easy-to measure, gettable and related

Goals with a deadline (SMART). Find out how turning your goals into easy-to-do

Parts raises enthusiasm and wins.

Celebrating Milestones

Enjoy small wins on your trip. Recognize and celebrate your successes, whether

It's learning a tough Pilate's exercise or reaching certain weight loss goals.

Tracking Progress

Keeping a Pilates Journal

Discover how keeping a Pilate's journal can help you follow your workouts,

Victories and struggles. Thinking about how far you've come makes you feel proud

And gives important clues in your exercise adventure.

Measurement beyond Weight

Use different ways to measure your progress that don't involve just the scale. Look At how strong, stretchy and fit you are as signs of success. This helps show a Complete picture of your workout accomplishments.

Overcoming Challenges

Embracing Mindfulness

Develop awareness in your Pilates work. Learn ways to focus during workouts, This will help you connect your mind and body better. This can make it easier for You to clear mental barriers.

Seeking Support

Make a group of friends or family that can help when things are tough. Having pals At the gym, online friends or expert help can give us encouragement and make sure We stick to our workout plans.

Making it Enjoyable

Variety in Workouts

Add different activities to your Pilates practice. Try out different types of

Exercises, change how you do them or go to new Pilate's classes. This will keep

Your workouts fun and exciting.

Adding Music and Slow Breathing to Mindfulness Practices

Make your Pilates better by adding music and careful breathing. Make lists of songs

That make you happy, and match your breath with movements to bring peace and joy into doing them.

Adapting to Changes

Flexibility in Routine

Learn why it's essential to have a flexible schedule for your exercise plan. Accept

Changes and adjustments when needed, which allows for a lasting way to keep doing

Your Pilates.

Periodic Assessments and Adjustments

Check your goals often and change how you work on them as needed. Know when

You need to make your workouts harder, add new tasks or change your food plan so

Tips for Safe and Effective Wall Pilates

Keeping safety and working well is very important in your Wall Pilates practice. This part gives tips, ways and ideas to help you get the most from your exercise While keeping harm low.

Listening to Your Body

Tuning into Sensations

Work on getting better at feeling sensations during your Pilates sessions. Learn the Difference between being uncomfortable and feeling pain, and change or fix Exercises if needed.

The significance of rest days

Recognize the importance of stopping and resting in your daily activities. Give your

Body time to regain strength and restore itself. This stops you from doing too much Exercise all at once, keeping a lasting practice in Pilates balanced for the long run.

Common Errors and How to Stay Clear of Them.

Proper Alignment Awareness

When doing exercises, remember to have the body in good position. Find out about

Typical mistakes in lining up and how to fix them so you don't hurt your joints or

Muscles.

Gradual Progression

Start with the easy things and then move to harder tasks. Don't try to do hard moves

Before you know basic ones. This will help keep you safe from getting hurt.

Seeking Professional Guidance

Certified Pilates Instructors

If you're new to Wall Pilates, think about working with a person who teaches it

Properly. They can help guide and instruct even beginners in the right way to practice this exercise method. Getting help from experts makes sure you use good form,

Changes things to fit you better and has a plan just for your goals in fitness.

Physical Health Consultation

Talk to a health expert before you start exercising, especially if you have medical

Problems or worries. This will help make sure your body is okay for the new exercise

Plan.

Using Proper Equipment

Quality Wall Surfaces

Pick safe and solid walls for your Pilates workout. Make sure the wall doesn't have

Anything in its way and gives enough help during workouts.

Appropriate Resistance Levels

When you use things like resistance bands, pick the right amount of power so your

Muscles don't get hurt. Slowly make it harder as you get stronger.

Incorporating Modifications

Adapting Movements

Practice changing your activities according to how fit you are and any problems with

Movement. Pilates has many changes so it can match different needs. This helps
Make the exercise better for everyone.

Individualizing Your Routine

Understand that each person's body is different. Make your Pilates exercise plan to
Fit with what you are good at and bad at, as well as the health goals you have.

Consistent Focus on Breath

Breathe Control Techniques

Focus on your breath regularly. Include breathing exercises in every exercise to
Improve air intake, strengthening core muscles and overall body-mind link.

Mindful Breathing during Challenges

When doing difficult exercises, remember to breathe slowly and carefully. This not
Only helps your physical work but also makes it easier to deal with stress and
Improves all of your Pilates activities.

Conclusion

On the last pages of "Wall Pilates Transformation", we ask you to think about not Just Emma's change but also what your chances are for improving yourself. You have a chance to live better and stronger as she did with her work out after wall hanging exercises in this book by me, (Doris A. Freema). This book is not just about Wall Pilates; it shows how powerful we all are to change our stories, make our bodies feel better and get more excited for a healthier life.

Emma went through the hard part of life today. It showed how difficult everything is – people being busy, getting angry with ordinary fitness plans and wanting a long lasting change that lasts. This happened to everyone including her too! By ending her story, we show that what she went through isn't just hers but is also faced by many others. This book is a way of saying that we all want fitness methods that not only work but also match how our lives really are.

When we say goodbye to Emma's story, we also ask you kindly - a fresh request for you to try Wall Pilates. It can change things in your life and make them better! Beyond these words, there is a chance for you to change personally. It's an Opportunity to start a new part of your own health story. This result isn't the end but

A start, telling you to use what you have learned and apply it in your everyday life. While losing weight is a big part of doing Wall Pilates, the end result shows it's much more than just physical changes. This book makes us change our view - a full picture way of feeling good that covers clear mind, strong feelings and new energy. The last

Parts say that being healthier is not just about losing weight, but also getting back your love for life.

As you finish the book, think of it as a last part in your own story. What will your fitness story look like in the future? How will Wall Pilates become a key part of your story about being healthy and feeling good? The finish makes you the writer of your ever-lasting trip. It gives you knowledge, motivation and tools found in these pages to help along the way.

In saying goodbye, we are very thankful that you joined us on this big journey. Your trip is special, and we are honored to have been involved in it. When you finish reading "Wall Pilates Transformation," take its energy into your every day. Use each new morning as a chance to grow, be strong and find happiness.

Happy New Starts and Long-lasting Changes!

With heartfelt gratitude,

Doris A. Freema

Your opinion matters

If you liked the good story, found it helpful or life changed a bit from what was written in it; please leave your thoughts about these changes on Amazon, Goodreads and other places where you looked at books. Help more people discover this book by showing them how great of publishing is done there with reviews:

Your review can be a couple of sentences talking about your whole experience, special parts you liked or how the book changed the way you think about staying fit and being healthy.

We know your time is important to you, and we really like any comments or suggestions you can give us. Thanks for being part of our group and thinking about

Sharing your ideas on "Wall Pilates Transformation."

I hope you keep succeeding in your journey to stay healthy!

Warm regards,

Doris A. Freema